Preface

Through the years of working as practitioner of energy medicine, I have come to my own technique regarding the wonderful tapping solutions to rebalance the energy flow in human emotions.

Here is a compact yet well-sorted collection of the frequently used techniques I have discovered and applied on my clients on their journey to self-help energetically. As reader, you are free to test these easy-to-use techniques for the well-being of yourself and those you care about.

In well-being,

Jessie Gao
December, 2013
Sweden

Introduction on Tapping Solution Á La Jessie

By working with my clients on diverse life issues, I have come to a more direct and simple-to-use meridian tapping technique which brings a faster energetic shift of emotional state of being.

Our personal realities are based on our individual interpretations about the world we live in and the events that affect our lives. The emotional energy that accumulates in our meridians creates and defines our emotional state of being and forms thereafter our personal worlds that we experience. This state of being is variable.

While tapping on selected meridians, we are empowered to renew our emotional energy with more harmony, comfort and ease, which leads to a natural and profound well-being. Now let's start to tap!

Content

1. How to tap against worry

∞

Step 1: the reasons behind worries

The human mind is often trapped by worry in front of the unknown and the uncertain.

However, we may not want to go and watch a football match should we already know the result in advance. Life on earth is a fascinating adventure, full of surprises and excitements.

Despite the illusion of man-made human worries, the universe continues to play its own game of change, expansion and growth.

- Before starting tapping, say calmly to yourself:

    Right now I am deeply worried about ... (my health, my job, my income, my family, my future, the global economy & environment, etc.)

Step 2: the desire for release from worries

Affirmations for the renewed inner state of feeling:

- It would be nice to feel more certainty ...

- It would be lovely to relax into ease ...

- It would be pleasant to let go with trust in life...

    Sit with upright back and relax with a few deep breaths to get ready for the tapping that follows.

    It works equally well with mental tapping in silence should you need to do so.

Step 3: energy renewal by tapping

Tap gently on the chest area (the area for heart chakra, stomach meridian and kidney meridian) with one hand (either with whole palm or five fingers);

Tap gently around the eyes (bladder meridian, gallbladder meridian, triple warmer meridian, stomach meridian) with fingers;

Tap gently with 3 fingers (forefinger, long finger and index finger) on the inside on the wrist (lung meridian, pericardium meridian and heart meridian) of the other hand.

At the same time use the following affirmations along your tapping:

- Even though I feel some worry inside of me right now, I can still choose to take it easy and enjoy a few deep breaths;

- Even though I am not sure about what's going to happen, I can still choose to give myself a break and to relax for a moment;

- Even though I feel uncertain about ... (my health, my job, my relation, etc.), I can still choose to shift my focus to something else for a moment and let the universe take over my worry now.

Repeat this set of affirmation 3-5 rounds with short breaks in between, when you take a few deep breaths to relax your mind and body.

Then go back to the initial feeling of worry and feel whether it has shifted into a feeling of ease.

If necessary, repeat a few more rounds of tapping till you sense a stronger shift of energy flow.

2. How to tap against fear & phobia

∞

Step 1: the reasons behind fear & phobia

The experiences of fear & phobia often occur upon the uncontrollable situations.

How would you feel if you reclaim your power to control the situation? There will be no more fear!

Fear drains your energy and takes you away from the true power you possess within. As co-creator of the universe, you come into life for the fearless adventure.

- Before starting tapping, say calmly to yourself:

  Right now I am bothered by my fear for ... (sickness, old age, death, pain, suffering, poverty, financial insecurity, break-down of love relationship, darkness, loneliness, height, crowd, spider, snake, water, noise, etc.)

Step 2: the desire for release from fear

Affirmations for the renewal of inner state of feeling:

- It would be nice to feel more calm ...

- It would be lovely to relax into security ...

- It would be pleasant to take actions with confidence ...

  Sit with upright back and relax with a few deep breaths to get ready for the tapping that follows.

  It works equally well with mental tapping in silence should you need to do so.

Step 3: energy renewal by tapping

Tap gently on the chest area (the area for heart chakra, stomach meridian and kidney meridian) with one hand (either with whole palm or five fingers);

Tap gently around the eyes (bladder meridian, gallbladder meridian, triple warmer meridian, stomach meridian) with fingers;

Tap gently with 3 fingers (forefinger, long finger and index finger) on the inside on the wrist (lung meridian, pericardium meridian and heart meridian) of the other hand.

At the same time use the following affirmations along your tapping:

- Even though I feel terrible fear inside of me right now, I can still choose to be a bit kinder to myself and take a few deep breaths;

- Even though I can't control over my emotions for invisible dangers, I can still allow myself to accept who I am;

- Even though I feel overwhelmed right now by my fear for ... (sickness, lack of money, losing the person I love, being alone, the terrible nervousness thinking about snakes, speaking in front of public, etc.), I can still choose to shift my focus to something else for a moment and take it easy with what's going on.

Repeat this set of affirmation 3-5 rounds with short breaks in between, when you take a few deep breaths to relax your mind and body.

Then go back to the initial feeling of fear and feel whether it has shifted into a feeling of ease.

If necessary, repeat a few more rounds of tapping till you sense a stronger shift of energy flow.

3. How to tap against anger & frustration

∞

Step 1: the reasons behind anger & frustration

Anger & frustration come to our experiences when we are run over by the unexpected events and don't know what to do with the current situation.

How would you feel if you have choices of solutions dealing with your situation? There will be no more anger or frustration!

Anger attacks you with high energy and makes you lose your common sense easily. In worst case, it can drive you crazy without orientation.

- Before starting tapping, say calmly to yourself:

Right now I am frustrated or angry about ... (my own behavior, the words and deeds of others, the injustice I witness, how I am treated by others, the silly reactions of others around me, etc.)

Step 2: the desire for release from anger

Affirmations for the renewal of inner state of feeling:

- It would be nice to feel more calm inside ...

- It would be lovely to relax into peace ...

- It would be pleasant to take actions with style ...

Sit with upright back and relax with a few deep breaths to get ready for the tapping that follows.

It works equally well with mental tapping in silence should you need to do so.

Step 3: energy renewal by tapping

Tap gently on the chest area (the area for heart chakra, stomach meridian and kidney meridian) with one hand (either with whole palm or five fingers);

Tap gently around the eyes (bladder meridian, gallbladder meridian, triple warmer meridian, stomach meridian) with fingers;

Tap gently with 3 fingers (forefinger, long finger and index finger) on the inside on the wrist (lung meridian, pericardium meridian and heart meridian) of the other hand.

At the same time use the following affirmations along your tapping:

- Even though I feel frustrated and angry right now, I can still choose to be a bit patient to myself and allow things to run its own course for a while;

- Even though I am not pleased with what's happening right now, I can still choose to give myself a moment and relax with a few deep breaths;

- Even though I feel overwhelmed right now by my anger about ... (the silly things that happen around me, the people who mistreat me, etc.), I can still choose to shift my focus to something else for a moment and accept myself as who I am.

Repeat this set of affirmation 3-5 rounds with short breaks in between, when you take a few deep breaths to relax your mind and body.

Then go back to the initial feeling of anger and feel whether it has shifted into a feeling of ease.

If necessary, repeat a few more rounds tapping till you sense a stronger shift of energy flow.

4. **How to tap against sorrow**

∞

Step 1: the reasons behind sorrow

Sorrow is caused by the feeling of lose. It triggers the inner conflict of wanting without holding. However, as eternal energy, each one of us is here on a temporary journey for the excitement of adventure. Nobody owns anything or anyone. Therefore, from a broader perspective there is no need to wipe in sorrow for anything.

Overwhelming sorrow lowers your energy dramatically, which affects negatively your daily performances in all aspects.

- Before starting tapping, say calmly to yourself:

Right now I feel deep sorrow for ... (the passing away of my loved ones, the natural disasters on earth, the sufferings of those I care, etc.)

Step 2: the desire for release from sorrow

Affirmations for the renewal of inner state of feeling:

- It would be nice to feel more calm now ...

- It would be lovely to relax into peace ...

- It would be pleasant to rest my mind with understanding ...

  Sit with upright back and relax with a few deep breaths to get ready for the tapping that follows.

  It works equally well with mental tapping in silence should you need to do so.

Step 3: energy renewal by tapping

Tap gently on the chest area (the area for heart chakra, stomach meridian and kidney meridian) with one hand (either with whole palm or five fingers);

Tap gently around the eyes (bladder meridian, gallbladder meridian, triple warmer meridian, stomach meridian) with fingers;

Tap gently with 3 fingers (forefinger, long finger and index finger) on the inside on the wrist (lung meridian, pericardium meridian and heart meridian) of the other hand.

At the same time use the following affirmations along your tapping:

- Even though I feel deep sorrow right now, I can still choose to be a bit kinder to myself and accept who I am completely;

- Even though I am not in control of the outer situations and changes, I can still choose to give myself a moment to relax and take a few deep breaths;

- Even though I feel overwhelmed right now by my sorrow for ... (the terrible things that have happened, the passing away of those I love, etc.), I can still choose to shift my focus to something else for a moment and accept myself as who I am.

Repeat this set of affirmation 3-5 rounds with short breaks in between, when you take a few deep breaths to relax your mind and body.

Then go back to the initial feeling of sorrow and feel whether it has shifted into a feeling of ease.

If necessary, repeat a few more rounds tapping till you sense a stronger shift of energy flow.

5. How to tap against depression

∞

Step 1: the reasons behind depression

Depression is the most common human emotion upon the loss of power over one's own life. In depression, one feels inadequate to deal with his or her own life in a satisfying manner.

Overwhelming depression empties your energy rapidly and leaves an empty space to fill, which often leads to very destructive thoughts such as suicide.

- Before starting tapping, say calmly to yourself:

  Right now I feel depressed for ... (the dark winter, the bad business I run, the broken family of mine, my hopeless future, my meaningless life, etc.)

Step 2: the desire for release from depression

Affirmations for the renewal of inner state of feeling:

- It would be nice to feel more energy inside ...

- It would be lovely to relax into hope ...

- It would be pleasant to take actions with new dreams and directions ...

Sit with upright back and relax with a few deep breaths to get ready for the tapping that follows.

It works equally well with mental tapping in silence should you need to do so.

Step 3: energy renewal by tapping

Tap gently on the chest area (the area for heart chakra, stomach meridian and kidney meridian) with one hand (either with whole palm or five fingers);

Tap gently around the eyes (bladder meridian, gallbladder meridian, triple warmer meridian, stomach meridian) with fingers;

Tap gently with 3 fingers (forefinger, long finger and index finger) on the inside on the wrist (lung meridian, pericardium meridian and heart meridian) of the other hand.

At the same time use the following affirmations along your tapping:

- Even though I feel deep depression right now, I can still choose to be more patient to myself and accept completely who I am;

- Even though I am not in the best form of myself, I can still choose to give myself a bit more time just to relax without doing anything;

- Even though I feel overwhelmed right now by my depression for ... (the disappointing performance of myself or others, the hopeless situation in my life, etc.), I can still choose to shift my focus to something else for a moment and accept myself as who I am.

Repeat this set of affirmation 3-5 rounds with short breaks in between, when you take a few deep breaths to relax your mind and body.

Then go back to the initial feeling of depression and feel whether it has shifted into a feeling of ease.

If necessary, repeat a few more rounds tapping till you sense a stronger shift of energy flow.

6. How to tap against stress

∞

Step 1: the reasons behind stress

Stress is the very most common mental challenge that mankind is faced in our modern world today. In spite of the advanced technology and security devices that make our living more convenient and efficient, deep inside we experience more tension than ever before. Fight-or-flee reflex has shifted into a severe mental battle, where we have to constantly figure out new ways to cope with new challenges of all kinds.

The overloading stress in our mind and body shuts the door to constructive thinking in ease. When overloaded by stress, we tend to make irrational decisions that cost us extra time, energy, money, and even worse our precious health...

- Before starting tapping, say calmly to yourself:

Right now I'm stressed for ... (my vacation plan, my dead-line at work, my exams in school, my family issues, my money problem, etc.)

Step 2: the desire for release from stress

Affirmations for the renewal of inner state of feeling:

- It would be nice to feel more relaxed now ...

- It would be lovely to rest into ease ...

- It would be pleasant to take actions with solid and reasonable solutions ...

   Sit with upright back and relax with a few deep breaths to get ready for the tapping that follows.

   It works equally well with mental tapping in silence should you need to do so.

Step 3: energy renewal by tapping

Tap gently on the chest area (the area for heart chakra, stomach meridian and kidney meridian) with one hand (either with whole palm or five fingers);

Tap gently around the eyes (bladder meridian, gallbladder meridian, triple warmer meridian, stomach meridian) with fingers;

Tap gently with 3 fingers (forefinger, long finger and index finger) on the inside on the wrist (lung meridian, pericardium meridian and heart meridian) of the other hand.

At the same time use the following affirmations along your tapping:

- Even though I feel very stressed right now, I can still choose to be more gentle to myself and accept completely who I am;

- Even though I am not in total harmony with myself, I can still choose to take a few deep breaths and relax for a while;

- Even though I feel overwhelmed right now by my stress for ... (the pressure at work and school, my family situations, money issues, and my future, etc.), I can still choose to shift my focus to something else for a moment and accept myself as who I am.

Repeat this set of affirmation 3-5 rounds with short breaks in between, when you take a few deep breaths to relax your mind and body.

Then go back to the initial feeling of depression and feel whether it has shifted into a feeling of ease.

If necessary, repeat a few more rounds tapping till you sense a stronger shift of energy flow.

7. How to tap against anxiety

∞

Step 1: the reasons behind anxiety

Rushing through life, many of us experience an uncontrollable anxiety in front of so-called big decisions to make. The harder we try, the harder the resistance we may create and the deeper anxiety is to be experienced.

Anxiety hurts and damages our inner peace and affects our common senses. We must understand that it takes time for things to develop in the direction we have designed. Therefore, it's reasonable to prepare yourself for the unexpected situations with calm spirit.

- Before starting tapping, say calmly to yourself:

Right now I feel anxiety regarding ... (my business, my job, my relations, my future, my money situation, my family issues, etc.)

Step 2: the desire for release from anxiety

Affirmations for the renewal of inner state of feeling:

- It would be nice to feel more collected within ...

- It would be lovely to relax into a peaceful mind ...

- It would be pleasant to take actions with smaller plans step by step ...

Sit with upright back and relax with a few deep breaths to get ready for the tapping that follows.

It works equally well with mental tapping in silence should you need to do so.

Step 3: energy renewal by tapping

Tap gently on the chest area (the area for heart chakra, stomach meridian and kidney meridian) with one hand (either with whole palm or five fingers);

Tap gently around the eyes (bladder meridian, gallbladder meridian, triple warmer meridian, stomach meridian) with fingers;

Tap gently with 3 fingers (forefinger, long finger and index finger) on the inside on the wrist (lung meridian, pericardium meridian and heart meridian) of the other hand.

At the same time use the following affirmations along your tapping:

- Even though I feel uncomfortable anxiety right now, I can still choose to be easier and kinder to myself and accept completely who I am;

- Even though I am not in total harmony with myself, I can still choose to give myself permission to take a break from trying;

- Even though I feel overwhelmed right now by my anxiety for ... (the serious decisions I have to make, the tough situations at work or in school, the conflicts at home, etc.), I can still choose to shift my focus to something else for a moment and accept myself completely as who I am.

Repeat this set of affirmation 3-5 rounds with short breaks in between, when you take a few deep breaths to relax your mind and body.

Then go back to the initial feeling of depression and feel whether it has shifted into a feeling of ease.

If necessary, repeat a few more rounds tapping till you sense a stronger shift of energy flow.

8. How to tap against low self-esteem

∞

Step 1: the reasons behind low self-esteem

Low self-esteem is a by-product of our inadequate understanding of who we really are. So often we are programmed as worthy only in relation to what we have done or how others judge ourselves. However, the infinite intelligence of creation sees no difference between our backgrounds or personalities, neither our human attributes we may carry. True worth of your existence is always guaranteed into eternity.

Low self-esteem blocks completely our natural creativity. All outstanding personalities and individuals through history share one attribute in common, which is powerful self-confidence and self-reliance.

- Before starting tapping, say calmly to yourself:

Right now I feel low self-esteem regarding ... (my school, my business, my job, my relations, my future, etc.)

Step 2: the desire for release from low self-esteem

Affirmations for the renewal of inner state of feeling:

- It would be nice to feel more self-certain inside ...

- It would be lovely to relax and enjoy my self-confidence...

- It would be pleasant to take actions with inner knowing of my true power ...

   Sit with upright back and relax with a few deep breaths to get ready for the tapping that follows.

   It works equally well with mental tapping in silence should you need to do so.

Step 3: energy renewal by tapping

Tap gently on the chest area (the area for heart chakra, stomach meridian and kidney meridian) with one hand (either with whole palm or five fingers);

Tap gently around the eyes (bladder meridian, gallbladder meridian, triple warmer meridian, stomach meridian) with fingers;

Tap gently with 3 fingers (forefinger, long finger and index finger) on the inside on the wrist of the other hand.

At the same time use the following affirmations along your tapping:

- Even though I feel terrible low self-esteem right now, I can still choose to be kinder to myself and accept completely who I am;

- Even though I am not confident about myself, I can still choose to allow myself to take it easy with everything around me;

- Even though I feel overwhelmed right now by my low self-esteem regarding ... (my performance in school or at work, my ability to earn more money, my desire for a love relation, my success to achieve my goals, etc.), I can still choose to shift my focus to something else for a moment and accept myself completely as who I am.

Repeat this set of affirmation 3-5 rounds with short breaks in between, when you take a few deep breaths to relax your mind and body.

Then go back to the initial feeling of depression and feel whether it has shifted into a feeling of ease.

If necessary, repeat a few more rounds tapping till you sense a stronger shift of energy flow.

9. How to tap against guilt & regret

∞

Step 1: the reasons behind guilt & regret

Guilt and regret belong to the first reactions upon our mistakes. The inner longing for being the best version of ourselves sometimes makes us disappointed when our performances don't meet our expectations. However, guilt & regret can't automatically inspire us into a constructive solution. For the purpose of self-improvement, we need focus our energy on the new targets and choices ahead.

Energetically, the emotion of guild & regret lowers our self-respect. Life is a great school full of various lessons and subjects. On the way of eternity, there is always one more step to take.

- Before starting tapping, say calmly to yourself:

Right now I feel guilt & regret regarding ... (my words or deeds, my decisions on business plan, my reactions toward those I care, etc.)

Step 2: the desire for release from guilt & regret

Affirmations for the renewal of inner state of feeling:

- It would be nice to feel more self-respect now ...

- It would be lovely to relax into self-forgiveness ...

- It would be pleasant to take actions with new perspective and insights ...

  Sit with upright back and relax with a few deep breaths to get ready for the tapping that follows.

  It works equally well with mental tapping in silence should you need to do so.

<u>Step 3: energy renewal by tapping</u>

Tap gently on the chest area (the area for heart chakra, stomach meridian and kidney meridian) with one hand (either with whole palm or five fingers);

Tap gently around the eyes (bladder meridian, gallbladder meridian, triple warmer meridian, stomach meridian) with fingers;

Tap gently with 3 fingers (forefinger, long finger and index finger) on the inside on the wrist (lung meridian, pericardium meridian and heart meridian) of the other hand.

At the same time use the following affirmations along your tapping:

- Even though I feel terrible guilt & regret right now, I can still choose to be kinder to myself and accept completely who I am;

- Even though I am not so proud of myself and my deeds right now, I can still choose to give myself permission to take a few deep breaths;

- Even though I feel overwhelmed right now by my guilt & regret for ... (saying the improper words to those I care, my careless business decisions, my immature attitude towards my mates and family members, etc.), I can still choose to shift my focus to something else for a moment and accept myself completely as who I am.

Repeat this set of affirmation 3-5 rounds with short breaks in between, when you take a few deep breaths to relax your mind and body.

Then go back to the initial feeling of depression and feel whether it has shifted into a feeling of ease.

If necessary, repeat a few more rounds tapping till you sense a stronger shift of energy flow.

10. How to tap against jealousy & hatred

∞

Step 1: the reasons behind jealousy & hatred

Unsatisfied desires often cause human jealousy & hatred. No matter how unfair it may appear on the surface, life does give us different kinds of gifts to fit our personal levels of awareness.

Being a unique being, each one of us has a unique position and value of our own, regardless of our social status. All inner organs must work in harmony to achieve a healthy body, so is it with our various personal talents and skills. There is no need to compare for the purpose of judgment.

- Before starting tapping, say calmly to yourself:

  Right now I feel jealousy & hatred about ... (the extra money of my neighbor, the extreme success of my old friends, the good luck of my colleges, the fancy stuff others possess, etc.)

Step 2: the desire for release from jealousy & hatred

Affirmations for the renewal of inner state of feeling:

- It would be nice to feel self-appreciation within ...

- It would be lovely to relax into self-satisfaction ...

- It would be pleasant to take actions with my own goals and allow others to have their goals too ...

Sit with upright back and relax with a few deep breaths to get ready for the tapping that follows.

It works equally well with mental tapping in silence should you need to do so.

Step 3: energy renewal by tapping

Tap gently on the chest area (the area for heart chakra, stomach meridian and kidney meridian) with one hand (either with whole palm or five fingers);

Tap gently around the eyes (bladder meridian, gallbladder meridian, triple warmer meridian, stomach meridian) with fingers;

Tap gently with 3 fingers (forefinger, long finger and index finger) on the inside on the wrist (lung meridian, pericardium meridian and heart meridian) of the other hand.

At the same time use the following affirmations along your tapping:

- Even though I feel terrible jealousy & hatred right now, I can still choose to be kinder to myself and accept completely who I am;

- Even though I am not totally satisfied of myself and my achievements right now, I can still choose to give myself permission to take a few deep breaths;

- Even though I feel overwhelmed right now by my jealousy & hatred for ... (the good luck of my neighbors, the huge money others have, the beauty of my classmates, the better jobs of my relatives, etc.), I can choose to shift my focus to something else for a moment and accept myself completely as who I am.

Repeat this set of affirmation 3-5 rounds with short breaks in between, when you take a few deep breaths to relax your mind and body.

Then go back to the initial feeling of depression and feel whether it has shifted into a feeling of ease.

If necessary, repeat a few more rounds tapping till you sense a stronger shift of energy flow.

11. How to tap against loneliness

∞

Step 1: the reasons behind loneliness

Human loneliness is often experienced when individuals feel disconnected to their inner source of contentment. Loneliness is an indication of our focus at the moment and is expected whenever a person focuses on illusion of separation from the universe.

As a co-creator of the universe, each one of us is always connected to the infinite power of the wholeness as water drops in a vast sea. We have constant communication with each other on different levels and dimensions, directly or indirectly.

- Before starting tapping, say calmly to yourself:

  Right now I feel a deep loneliness regarding ... (the empty home I live, the lonely night I have, the unfamiliar environment around me, the passing away of my loved ones, the misunderstanding of others, etc.)

Step 2: the desire for release from loneliness

Affirmations for the renewal of inner state of feeling:

- It would be nice to feel connected to life without separation...

- It would be lovely to relax into self-assurance ...

- It would be pleasant to focus on the infinite universe of unconditional guidance, support and blessings ...

Sit with upright back and relax with a few deep breaths to get ready for the tapping that follows.

It works equally well with mental tapping in silence should you need to do so.

Step 3: energy renewal by tapping

Tap gently on the chest area (the area for heart chakra, stomach meridian and kidney meridian) with one hand (either with whole palm or five fingers);

Tap gently around the eyes (bladder meridian, gallbladder meridian, triple warmer meridian, stomach meridian) with fingers;

Tap gently with 3 fingers (forefinger, long finger and index finger) on the inside on the wrist (lung meridian, pericardium meridian and heart meridian) of the other hand.

At the same time use the following affirmations along your tapping:

- Even though I feel a deep loneliness right now, I can still choose to be gentle to myself and accept completely who I am;

- Even though I am not totally connected to my own true nature right now, I can still choose to give myself some time to take it easy;

- Even though I feel overwhelmed right now by my unbearable loneliness caused by ... (the passing away of my loved ones, the lost job I needed, the misunderstandings around me, etc.), I can still choose to shift my focus to something else for a moment and accept myself unconditionally.

Repeat this set of affirmation 3-5 rounds with short breaks in between, when you take a few deep breaths to relax your mind and body.

Then go back to the initial feeling of depression and feel whether it has shifted into a feeling of ease.

If necessary, repeat a few more rounds tapping till you sense a stronger shift of energy flow.

12. How to tap against trauma

∞

Step 1: the reasons behind trauma

The experience of trauma is caused by unexpected events which appear as a shock to the human mind. The drama of life is eager to show us various scenes of human interplays, some of which leave a mark of unexpected trauma in the mind.

Trauma damages our integrity if we are powerless to deal with it. Tapping empowers you with a powerful tool for self-help and self-healing.

- Before starting tapping, say calmly to yourself:

  Right now I feel very uncomfortable thinking about the trauma I have experienced caused by ... (the war memories, the family conflicts, the mistreatments in my childhood, etc.)

Step 2: the desire for release from trauma

Affirmations for the renewal of inner state of feeling:

- It would be nice to feel calm & collected inside ...

- It would be lovely to relax into peaceful mind ...

- It would be pleasant to focus on new solutions to re-establish my integrity in life ...

Sit with upright back and relax with a few deep breaths to get ready for the tapping that follows.

It works equally well with mental tapping in silence should you need to do so.

Step 3: energy renewal by tapping

Tap gently on the chest area (the area for heart chakra, stomach meridian and kidney meridian) with one hand (either with whole palm or five fingers);

Tap gently around the eyes (bladder meridian, gallbladder meridian, triple warmer meridian, stomach meridian) with fingers;

Tap gently with 3 fingers (forefinger, long finger and index finger) on the inside on the wrist (lung meridian, pericardium meridian and heart meridian) of the other hand.

At the same time use the following affirmations along your tapping:

- Even though I feel a chaotic trauma inside of me right now, I can still take a few deep breaths to be kind to myself with acceptance of who I am;

- Even though I am deeply bothered by my inner chaos & trauma, I can still choose to allow myself to take it easy right now;

- Even though I feel overwhelmed right now by my terrible trauma caused by ... (the painful war memories, the bitter experiences in my school time, the harsh treatment by my family, my shocking witness of traffic accidents, etc.), I can still choose to shift my focus to something else for a moment and accept myself unconditionally.

Repeat this set of affirmation 3-5 rounds with short breaks in between, when you take a few deep breaths to relax your mind and body.

Then go back to the initial feeling of depression and feel whether it has shifted into a feeling of ease.

If necessary, repeat a few more rounds tapping till you sense a stronger shift of energy flow.

3

Epilogue

Tapping technique is one of the most up-to-date and easy-to-use techniques for self-help & self-healing, as well as a remarkable appliance of the TCM (traditional Chinese medicine) in the field of personal development of our modern time.

Tap often, tap with focus, tap creatively, and tap into the best emotional balance which benefits yourself and all others you get in touch with.

Good luck! ☺